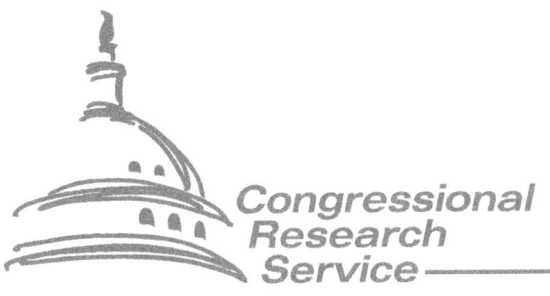

Title X (Public Health Service Act) Family Planning Program

Angela Napili
Information Research Specialist

August 28, 2012

Congressional Research Service
7-5700
www.crs.gov
RL33644

CRS Report for Congress
Prepared for Members and Committees of Congress

Summary

The federal government provides grants for voluntary family planning services through the Family Planning Program, Title X of the Public Health Service Act (42 U.S.C. §§ 300 to 300a-6). Enacted in 1970, it is the only domestic federal program devoted solely to family planning and related preventive health services. Title X is administered through the Office of Population Affairs (OPA) in the Department of Health and Human Services (HHS). Although the authorization of appropriations for Title X ended with FY1985, funding for the program has continued through appropriations bills for the Departments of Labor, Health and Human Services, and Education, and Related Agencies (Labor-HHS-Education).

FY2012 funding for Title X is $293.870 million, 2% less than the FY2011 funding level of $299.400 million. The Consolidated Appropriations Act, 2012 (P.L. 112-74) continues previous years' requirements that Title X funds not be spent on abortions, that all pregnancy counseling be nondirective, and that funds not be spent on promoting or opposing any legislative proposal or candidate for public office. Grantees continue to be required to certify that they encourage "family participation" when minors seek family planning services, and certify that they counsel minors on how to resist attempted coercion into sexual activity. The law also clarifies that family planning providers are not exempt from state notification and reporting laws on child abuse, child molestation, sexual abuse, rape, or incest.

The President's FY2013 Budget requests $296.838 million for Title X, 1% more than the FY2012 funding level. The Senate-reported FY2013 Labor-HHS-Education Appropriations bill, S. 3295, would provide $293.870 million. The draft appropriations bill approved by the House Appropriations Subcommittee on Labor, Health and Human Services, Education, and Related Agencies would provide zero funding for Title X in FY2013.

The law (42 U.S.C. §300a-6) prohibits the use of Title X funds in programs where abortion is a method of family planning. According to OPA, family planning projects that receive Title X funds are closely monitored to ensure that federal funds are used appropriately and that funds are not used for prohibited activities such as abortion. The prohibition on abortion does not apply to all the activities of a Title X grantee, but only to activities that are part of the Title X project. A grantee's abortion activities must be "separate and distinct" from the Title X project activities.

Several bills addressing Title X have been introduced in the 112th Congress. H.R. 217 and S. 96 would prohibit Title X grants to abortion-performing entities. H.R. 408 and S. 178 would eliminate the Title X program. H.R. 1099 would prohibit federal spending on any family planning activity. H.R. 1135, H.R. 1167, and S. 1904 would require an overall spending limit on means-tested welfare programs, defined to include family planning. S. 814 would require online disclosure of audits conducted under Title X on any entity receiving Title X funds. H.R. 5650 would prohibit Title X grantees and contractors from discriminating against a health care entity on the basis of whether it separately provides or refers for abortions, provides employees coverage of abortions, or provides or requires training in performing abortions. H.R. 1 would have eliminated funding for Title X for FY2011. H.R. 1 and H.Con.Res. 36 would have restricted federal funding to the Planned Parenthood Federation of America (PPFA) and its affiliates for FY2011. The House-introduced FY2012 Labor-HHS-Education Appropriations bill, H.R. 3070, would have prohibited the bill's funds from being used for Title X. H.R. 3070 would have also restricted the bill's funding to PPFA and its affiliates unless they certify that the organization will not perform abortions.

Contents

Title X Program Administration and Grants 1
  Administration 1
  Family Planning Services Grants 1
    Services 1
      Client Charges 2
      Client Characteristics 2
      Grantees and Clinics 3
  Family Planning Training and Research Grants 3
FY2013 Funding 3
  Budget Request 3
  Senate Activity 4
  House Activity 5
  Continuing Resolution 5
FY2012 Funding 6
Institute of Medicine Evaluation 8
The Patient Protection and Affordable Care Act and Title X 10
Abortion and Title X 13
Teenage Pregnancy and Title X 15
Confidentiality for Minors and Title X 16
Planned Parenthood and Title X 17
Provider Conscience Rule 18
  Overview 18
  2008 Rule 19
  2011 Rule Rescission 20
Legislation in the 112th Congress 22
  Abortion Restrictions 22
  Elimination of Title X Funds 22
  Public Disclosure of Audits 23
  Nondiscrimination on the Basis of Abortion Provision with Non-Title X Funds 24
  Limits on Means-Tested Welfare Spending 24
  Restrictions on Funding to Planned Parenthood 24
  Maternity Care Home Demonstration 25
  HIV/AIDS Provider Loan Repayment Program 25

Tables

Table 1. Title X Family Planning Program Appropriations 8

Appendixes

Appendix. Summary of Title X of the Public Health Service Act 26

Contacts

Author Contact Information...27

Title X Program Administration and Grants

Administration

Title X is administered by the Office of Population Affairs' (OPA's) Office of Family Planning (OFP), under the Office of the Assistant Secretary for Health in the Department of Health and Human Services (HHS). Although the program is administered through OPA, funding for Title X activities is provided through the Health Resources and Services Administration (HRSA) in HHS. Authorization of appropriations expired at the end of FY1985, but the program has continued to be funded through appropriations bills for the Departments of Labor, Health and Human Services, and Education, and Related Agencies (Labor-HHS-Education).

OPA administers three types of project grants under Title X: family planning services;[1] family planning personnel training;[2] and family planning service delivery improvement research grants.[3]

Family Planning Services Grants

Services

Ninety percent of Title X funds are used for clinical services.[4] Grants for family planning services fund family planning and related preventive health services, such as natural family planning methods; infertility services; services to adolescents; breast and cervical cancer screening and prevention; sexually transmitted disease (STD) and HIV prevention education, counseling, testing, and referral; preconception counseling; and counseling on establishing a reproductive life plan. Among the program's FY2012 priorities is one for providing preventive health services "in accordance with nationally recognized standards of care."[5] The services must be provided "without coercion and with respect for the privacy, dignity, social, and religious beliefs of the individuals being served."[6]

Title X clinics provide confidential screening, counseling, and referral for treatment. In this regard, OPA has expressed a commitment to integrating HIV-prevention services in all family planning clinics.[7] OPA provides supplemental grants to help Title X projects implement the

---

[1] *Catalog of Federal Domestic Assistance (CFDA)*, Program number 93.217, http://www.cfda.gov.

[2] *CFDA*, Program number 93.260.

[3] *CFDA*, Program number 93.974.

[4] HHS, Health Resources and Services Administration, *Fiscal Year 2013 Justification of Estimates for Appropriations Committees*, p. 348, http://www.hrsa.gov/about/budget/budgetjustification2013.pdf.

[5] U.S. Department of Health and Human Services (HHS), Office of Population Affairs, *Fiscal Year 2012 Program Priorities*, http://www.hhs.gov/opa/title-x-family-planning/title-x-policies/program-priorities/. OPA also instructed providers that clinical protocols should reflect recognized standards of care in "OPA Program Instruction Series, OPA 09-01: Clinical Services in Title X Family Planning Clinics – Consistency with Current Practice Recommendations," letter from Evelyn M. Kappeler, acting director, Office of Population Affairs, to Regional Health Administrators, Regions I-X, April 28, 2009, http://www.hhs.gov/opa/title-x-family-planning/initiatives-and-resources/documents-and-tools/opa-09-01.html.

[6] *CFDA*, Program number 93.217. See also 42 C.F.R. §59.5.

[7] HHS, Office of Population Affairs (OPA), *HIV Prevention and Integration in Family Planning*, http://www.hhs.gov/opa/title-x-family-planning/initiatives-and-resources/hiv-prevention-and-integration/.

Centers for Disease Control and Prevention's "Revised Recommendations for HIV Testing of Adults, Adolescents, and Pregnant Women in Health Care Settings."[8]

Title X services offered to males include condoms, education and counseling, STD testing and treatment, HIV testing, and, in some cases, vasectomy services.[9]

Client Charges

Priority for services is given to persons from low-income families, who may not be charged for care.[10] Clients from families with income between 100% and 250% of the federal poverty guideline (FPL) are charged on a sliding scale based on their ability to pay. Clients from families with income higher than 250% FPL are charged fees designed to recover the reasonable cost of providing services.[11]

Client Characteristics

In 2010, Title X-funded clinics served 5.225 million clients, primarily low-income women and adolescents. Of those clients, 8% were male,[12] 69% had incomes at or below the federal poverty level, and 90% had incomes at or below 200% of the federal poverty level.[13] For more than half of clients, Title X clinics are their "usual" or only continuing source of health care.[14] In 2010, 67% of Title X clients were uninsured.[15]

---

[8] Centers for Disease Control and Prevention (CDC), "Revised Recommendations for HIV Testing of Adults, Adolescents, and Pregnant Women in Health-Care Settings," *MMWR Recommendations and Reports*, vol. 55, no. RR-14 (September 26, 2006), pp. 1-17, http://www.cdc.gov/mmwr/preview/mmwrhtml/rr5514a1.htm. See also CDC, *HIV Testing in Healthcare Settings*, http://www.cdc.gov/hiv/topics/testing/healthcare/.

[9] HHS, OPA/Office of Family Planning, *Male Services,* http://www.hhs.gov/opa/title-x-family-planning/initiatives-and-resources/male-services/.

[10] 42 C.F.R. §59.2 defines "low-income family" as having income at or below 100% of the Federal Poverty Guidelines (FPL). The regulation states that "'Low-income family' also includes members of families whose annual family income exceeds this amount, but who, as determined by the project director, are unable, for good reasons, to pay for family planning services. For example, unemancipated minors who wish to receive services on a confidential basis must be considered on the basis of their own resources."

[11] 42 C.F.R. §59.5.

[12] Christina Fowler, Stacey Lloyd, Julia Gable, Jiantong Wang, and Kathleen Krieger, *Family Planning Annual Report: 2010 National Summary*, RTI International, Research Triangle Park, NC, September 2011, pp. 8-9, http://www.hhs.gov/opa/pdfs/fpar-2010-national-summary.pdf.

[13] Christina Fowler, Stacey Lloyd, Julia Gable, Jiantong Wang, and Kathleen Krieger, *Family Planning Annual Report: 2010 National Summary*, p. 22.

[14] HHS, Health Resources and Services Administration, *Fiscal Year 2013 Justification of Estimates for Appropriations Committees*, p. 348. See also Figure 2.3, "The large majority of women who obtain care at a family planning center consider it their usual source of care," in Rachel Benson Gold, Adam Sonfield, and Cory L. Richards, et al., *Next Steps for America's Family Planning Program: Leveraging the Potential of Medicaid and Title X in an Evolving Health Care System*, Guttmacher Institute, New York, 2009, p. 14, http://www.guttmacher.org/pubs/NextSteps.pdf.

[15] Christina Fowler, Stacey Lloyd, Julia Gable, Jiantong Wang, and Kathleen Krieger, *Family Planning Annual Report: 2010 National Summary*, pp. 21, 23.

Grantees and Clinics

In 2010, there were 89 Title X family planning services grantees. Such grantees included 49 state, local, and territorial health departments and 40 nonprofit organizations, such as hospitals, community health centers, family planning councils, Planned Parenthood affiliates, and universities.[16]

Title X grantees can provide family planning services directly or they can delegate Title X monies to other agencies to provide services. Although there are no matching requirements for grants, regulations specify that no clinics may be fully supported by Title X funds.[17] In 2010, Title X provided services through 4,389 clinics located in the 50 states, the District of Columbia, and the U.S. territories.[18]

Family Planning Training and Research Grants

Grants for family planning personnel training are used to train staff and to improve the use and career development of paraprofessionals.[19] Staff are trained through 10 regional general training programs and 3 national training programs.[20] Family planning service delivery improvement research grants are used to develop studies to enhance effectiveness and efficiency of the service delivery system.

More information on the Title X program can be found at http://www.hhs.gov/opa/title-x-family-planning/.

FY2013 Funding

Budget Request

The President's FY2013 Budget requests $296.838 million for Title X. This would be a 1% increase over the FY2012 level of $293.870 million.[21] The budget would continue previous years' requirements that Title X funds not be spent on abortions, that all pregnancy counseling be nondirective, and that funds not be spent on promoting or opposing any legislative proposal or candidate for public office.[22]

---

[16] Christina Fowler, Stacey Lloyd, Julia Gable, Jiantong Wang, and Kathleen Krieger, *Family Planning Annual Report: 2010 National Summary*, p. 7.

[17] 42 C.F.R. §59.7(c).

[18] Christina Fowler, Stacey Lloyd, Julia Gable, Jiantong Wang, and Kathleen Krieger, *Family Planning Annual Report: 2010 National Summary*, p. 7. A searchable directory of Title X providers is at HHS, OPA, *Family Planning Clinic Updates*, https://opa-fpclinics.icfwebservices.com.

[19] *CFDA*, Program number 93.260.

[20] HHS, OPA, *Regional Training Centers*, http://www.hhs.gov/opa/title-x-family-planning/training/regional-training-centers/.

[21] HHS, HRSA, *Fiscal Year 2013, Justification of Estimates for Appropriations Committees*, p. 347.

[22] HHS, HRSA, *Fiscal Year 2013, Justification of Estimates for Appropriations Committees*, p. 19.

Highlights from the FY2013 HRSA Budget *Justification* include the following:

- The proposed FY2013 funding level is projected to support family planning services for 5 million clients.

- The program's FY2013 goals include preventing 1,600 cases of infertility through Chlamydia screening and 961,000 unintended pregnancies.

- Family planning clinics will be encouraged to use electronic health records and electronic practice management systems and to improve clinics' ability to bill third parties.

- The program will continue to try to increase competition for funds, targeting areas that currently lack access to family planning services.

- The program will continue to try to improve clinic efficiency in response to rising costs for pharmaceuticals, providers, and screening and diagnostic technologies.

- The FY2013 target for cost per client served is $292.23, with the goal of maintaining the cost per client below the medical care inflation rate.

- Clinics will be encouraged to expand the availability of long-acting reversible contraceptive methods.

- The FY2013 HRSA *Justification* describes plans to continue a contract with the Institute of Medicine (IOM) for a Standing Committee to advise the Title X program. The Standing Committee is examining the role of family planning and reproductive health in health reform and will address recommendations made in the independent IOM report, *A Review of the HHS Family Planning Program: Mission, Management, and Measurement of Results* (2009). (The IOM report is discussed further in the section "Institute of Medicine Evaluation.")[23]

Senate Activity

On June 14, 2012, the Senate Appropriations Committee approved its FY2013 Labor-HHS-Education appropriations bill, S. 3295. The bill would provide $293.870 million for Title X, the same as the FY2012 funding level.

S. 3295 would continue previous years' requirements that Title X funds not be spent on abortions, that all pregnancy counseling be nondirective, and that funds not be spent on "any activity (including the publication or distribution of literature) that in any way tends to promote public support or opposition to any legislative proposal or candidate for public office." Grantees would continue to be required to certify that they encourage "family participation" when minors decide to seek family planning services and that they counsel minors on how to resist attempted coercion into sexual activity. The bill also clarifies that family planning providers are not exempt from state notification and reporting laws on child abuse, child molestation, sexual abuse, rape, or incest.

In the committee report, the Senate Appropriations Committee supported updating program guidance to clarify that Title X funds may be used for information technology training and

---

[23] HHS, HRSA, *Fiscal Year 2013, Justification of Estimates for Appropriations Committees*, pp. 347-353.

implementation, including electronic medical records. The committee also directed HRSA and the HHS Secretary to take certain steps to allow Title X-funded specialized family planning centers to be National Health Service Corps (NHSC) sites.[24]

House Activity

On July 18, 2012, the House Appropriations Subcommittee on Labor, Health and Human Services, Education, and Related Agencies approved its draft FY2013 appropriations bill, which would prohibit the bill's funds from being used for the Title X program.[25]

The House subcommittee's draft bill would continue previous years' language requiring Title X grantees to certify that they encourage "family participation" when minors decide to seek family planning services and that they counsel minors on how to resist attempted coercion into sexual activity. The draft bill also clarifies that family planning providers are not exempt from state notification and reporting laws on child abuse, child molestation, sexual abuse, rape, or incest.

The House subcommittee's draft bill would prohibit the bill's funds from being made available "for any purpose" to the Planned Parenthood Federation of America (PPFA) or any of its affiliates and clinics, unless they certify that PPFA affiliates and clinics will not perform an abortion, and will not provide any funds to any other entity that performs an abortion. There are exceptions for rape, incest, and certain physician-certified cases in which the woman is "in danger of death unless an abortion is performed." The HHS Secretary would be required to "seek repayment of any Federal assistance received by Planned Parenthood Federation of America, Inc., or any affiliate or clinic of Planned Parenthood Federation of America, Inc., if it violates the terms of the certification required by this section."

Continuing Resolution

On July 31, 2012, House and Senate leaders announced a bipartisan agreement to consider a six-month FY2013 continuing resolution (CR). The CR would provide appropriations from October 2012 through March 2013. According to the announcements, the CR would be consistent with the spending cap in the Budget Control Act, which limits FY2013 federal discretionary spending to $1.047 trillion. The announcements did not specify program funding levels. The House and the Senate are expected to consider the continuing resolution in September 2012.[26]

---

[24] S.Rept. 112-176, pp. 56-57. NHSC sites are required to provide referrals to comprehensive primary care services. The Senate Appropriations Committee directed HRSA to align Title X's and NHSC's definitions of "comprehensive primary care services." The committee also directed the HHS Secretary to provide guidance to Title X-only funded grantees on how to meet NHSC site requirements. For discussion of NHSC issues, see Rachel Benson Gold, "The National Health Service Corps: An Answer to Family Planning Centers' Workforce Woes?," *Guttmacher Policy Review*, vol. 14, no. 1 (Winter 2011), pp. 11-15; and Adam Sonfield, "Washington Watch: Providers look to help from workforce program," *Contraceptive Technology Update*, July 1, 2011.

[25] U.S. Congress, House Committee on Appropriations, Subcommittee on Labor, Health and Human Services, Education, and Related Agencies, *Making appropriations for the Departments of Labor, Health and Human Services, and Education, and related agencies for the fiscal year ending September 30, 2012, and for other purposes*, Draft bill, 112th Cong., 2nd sess., July 15, 2012, Sections 208, 209, 219, and 536, http://appropriations.house.gov/uploadedfiles/bills-112hr-sc-ap-fy13-laborhhsed.pdf.

[26] Speaker of the House John Boehner, "Speaker Boehner: House & Senate to Pass Six-Month CR in September," press release, July 31, 2012, http://www.speaker.gov/press-release/speaker-boehner-house-senate-pass-six-month-cr-(continued...)

FY2012 Funding

FY2012 funding for Title X is $293.870 million, 2% less than the FY2011 level of $299.400 million.[27] P.L. 112-74, the Consolidated Appropriations Act, 2012, continues previous years' requirements that Title X funds not be spent on abortions, that all pregnancy counseling be nondirective, and that funds not be spent on "any activity (including the publication or distribution of literature) that in any way tends to promote public support or opposition to any legislative proposal or candidate for public office." Grantees continue to be required to certify that they encourage "family participation" when minors decide to seek family planning services and that they counsel minors on how to resist attempted coercion into sexual activity. The law also clarifies that family planning providers are not exempt from state notification and reporting laws on child abuse, child molestation, sexual abuse, rape, or incest.[28]

The Consolidated Appropriations Act, 2012, contains a clause, known as the Weldon Amendment, stating that "None of the funds made available in this Act may be made available to a Federal agency or program, or to a State or local government, if such agency, program, or government subjects any institutional or individual health care entity to discrimination on the basis that the health care entity does not provide, pay for, provide coverage of, or refer for abortions."[29] Some have argued that the Weldon Amendment conflicts with regulations that require Title X family planning services projects to give pregnant women the opportunity to receive information, counseling, and referral upon request for several options, including "pregnancy termination."[30] In

---

(...continued)

september. Senate Majority Leader Harry Reid, "Reid Announces Deal With House, White House To Fund Government Through First Quarter Of 2013," press release, July 31, 2012, http://www.reid.senate.gov/newsroom/pr_073112_reid-announces-government-funding-2013.cfm. For more background on the Budget Control Act, see CRS Report R41965, *The Budget Control Act of 2011*.

[27] HHS, Health Resources and Services Administration, *Fiscal Year 2013 Justification of Estimates for Appropriations Committees*, p. 347. The Consolidated Appropriations Act, 2012 (P.L. 112-74) at 125 Stat. 1066, initially provided $297.400 million for Title X in FY2012; Division F, Title V, section 527 applied a 0.189% across-the-board rescission to most Labor-HHS-Education items, bringing the funding level to $296.838 million (125 Stat. 1115). In January 2012, the HHS Secretary announced the transfer of $2.968 million from Title X to HIV/AIDS assistance programs, bringing the Title X funding level to $293.870 million (Letter from Kathleen Sebelius, Secretary of Health and Human Services, to the Honorable Tom Harkin, January 20, 2012). Prior to passage of the Consolidated Appropriations Act, 2012 (P.L. 112-74), Congress provided temporary FY2012 funding under three continuing resolutions. P.L. 112-33, the Continuing Appropriations Act, 2012, provided funding through October 4, 2011. P.L. 112-36, the Continuing Appropriations Act, 2012, provided funding through November 18, 2011. P.L. 112-55, the Consolidated and Further Continuing Appropriations Act, 2012, provided funding through December 16, 2011. For most federal programs, including Title X Family Planning, these continuing resolutions continued funding under the same authority and conditions as for FY2011, but with a 1.503% across-the-board reduction in the rate of operations.

[28] P.L. 112-74, Division F, Title II, §209 and §210.

[29] P.L. 112-74, Division F, §507(d). The Weldon Amendment was originally adopted as part of the FY2005 Labor-HHS-Education appropriations law, and has been attached to each subsequent Labor-HHS-Education appropriations law: P.L. 108-447, Division F, §508(d), 118 Stat. 3163 (FY2005); P.L. 109-149, §508(d), 119 Stat. 2879 (FY2006). Under P.L. 110-5, §2, 121 Stat. 8, FY2007 appropriations were subject to the same conditions as during FY2006. P.L. 110-161, Division G, §508(d), 121 Stat. 1844 (FY2008). P.L. 111-8, Division F, §508(d), 123 Stat. 803 (FY2009). P.L. 111-117, Division D, §508(d), 123 Stat. 3280 (FY2010). Under P.L. 112-10, Division B, §1101, FY2011 appropriations were subject to the same conditions as during FY2010.

[30] 42 C.F.R. 59.5(a)(5). Examples of this argument appear in "Weldon Amendment," *Congressional Record*, daily edition, vol. 151, no. 51 (April 25, 2005), p. S4222; and "Federal Refusal Clause," *Congressional Record*, daily edition, vol. 151, no. 52 (April 26, 2005), p. S425. The National Family Planning and Reproductive Health Association (NFPRHA), many of whose members provide Title X services, filed a lawsuit challenging the Weldon Amendment in the U.S. District Court for the District of Columbia. The court found that "While Weldon may not provide the level of (continued...)

the February 23, 2011, *Federal Register*, HHS stated of potential conflicts, "The approach of a case by case investigation and, if necessary, enforcement will best enable the Department to deal with any perceived conflicts within concrete situations."[31] This issue is discussed further in "Provider Conscience Rule" below.

On September 22, 2011, the Senate Appropriations Committee reported S. 1599, the Departments of Labor, Health and Human Services, and Education, and Related Agencies Appropriations Act, 2012. In the accompanying committee report S.Rept. 112-84, the Senate Appropriations Committee stated that it was aware of the 2009 Institute of Medicine review of the program, and that it supports the OFP's efforts to review and update Title X program guidance and administrative directives.[32] The committee also stated that it encourages HRSA to allocate resources to OPA from the Patient Protection and Affordable Care Act (ACA). These resources would be used for technical assistance to help grantees prepare for ACA implementation, "including the expansion of Medicaid, technology upgrades and participating essential community providers."[33]

(...continued)
guidance that NFPRHA or its members would prefer, may create a conflict with pre-existing agency regulations, and may impose conditions that NFPRHA members find unacceptable, none of these reasons provides a sufficient basis for the court to invalidate an act of Congress in its entirety." Upon appeal, the U.S. Court of Appeals for the District of Columbia Circuit found that the plaintiff lacked the standing to challenge the Weldon Amendment. *See National Family Planning and Reproductive Health Association, Inc., v. Alberto Gonzales, et al.*, 468 F.3d 826 (D.C. Cir. 2006), and 391 F. Supp. 2d 200, 209 (D.D.C. 2005).

[31] HHS, "Regulation for the Enforcement of Federal Health Care Provider Conscience Protection Laws," 76 *Federal Register* 9973, February 23, 2010.

[32] S.Rept. 112-84, p. 58.

[33] Beginning in 2014, ACA will provide certain individuals and small businesses with access to private health plans through new health insurance exchanges. To ensure access for low-income individuals, most exchange plans will be required to have a sufficient number and geographic distribution of "essential community providers," which include Title X projects. U.S. Health and Human Services Department, "Patient Protection and Affordable Care Act; Establishment of Exchanges and Qualified Health Plans; Exchange Standards for Employers," 77 *Federal Register* 18470, March 27, 2012; 45 C.F.R. § 156.235

Table 1. Title X Family Planning Program Appropriations
(in millions)

FY	Appropriation	FY	Appropriation	FY	Appropriation
1971	$6.0	1986	$136.4	2001	$253.9
1972	$61.8	1987	$142.5	2002	$265.0
1973	$100.6	1988	$139.7	2003	$273.4
1974	$100.6	1989	$138.3	2004	$278.3
1975	$100.6	1990	$139.1	2005	$286.0
1976	$100.6	1991	$144.3	2006	$282.9
1977	$113.0	1992	$149.6	2007	$283.1
1978	$135.0	1993	$173.4	2008	$300.0
1979	$135.0	1994	$180.9	2009	$307.5
1980	$162.0	1995	$193.3	2010	$317.5
1981	$161.7	1996	$192.6	2011	$299.4
1982	$124.2	1997	$198.5	2012	$293.9
1983	$124.1	1998	$203.5	2013	a
1984	$140.0	1999	$215.0		
1985	$142.5	2000	$238.9		

Source: FY1971-FY2005: Department of Health and Human Services, Office of Population Affairs, *Funding History*, http://www.hhs.gov/opa/title-x-family-planning/title-x-policies/title-x-funding-history/; FY2006: Senate Appropriations Committee, S.Rept. 109-287, p. 325; FY2007: *Consolidated Appropriations Act, 2008 Committee Print of the House Committee on Appropriations on H.R. 2764/P.L. 110-161*, p. 1793, http://www.gpo.gov/fdsys/pkg/CPRT-110HPRT39564; FY2008-FY2009: "Explanatory Statement Submitted by Mr. Obey, Chairman of the House Committee on Appropriations, Regarding H.R. 1105, Omnibus Appropriations Act, 2009," *Congressional Record*, daily edition, vol. 155, no. 31 (February 23, 2009), p. H2378. FY2010: P.L. 111-117, 123 Stat. 3239. FY2011: P.L. 112-10, §1810 and §1119. FY2012: HHS, HRSA, *Fiscal Year 2013 Justification of Estimates for Appropriations Committees*, p. 347.

a. The FY2013 funding level has not yet been finalized. The President's FY2013 Budget requests $296.8 million. The Senate-reported FY2013 Labor-HHS-Education Appropriations bill, S. 3295, proposes $293.9 million. The House Appropriations Labor-HHS-Education Subcommittee's draft FY2013 bill proposes zero funding for Title X.

Institute of Medicine Evaluation

At the request of OFP, the Institute of Medicine (IOM) of the National Academy of Sciences independently evaluated the Title X program and made recommendations in *A Review of the HHS Family Planning Program: Mission, Management, and Measurement of Results* (2009).[34]

---

[34] Institute of Medicine (IOM), Committee on a Comprehensive Review of the HHS Office of Family Planning Title X Program, *A Review of the HHS Family Planning Program: Mission, Management, and Measurement of Results*, ed. Adrienne Stith Butler and Ellen Wright Clayton (Washington, DC: The National Academies Press, 2009), http://www.nap.edu/catalog.php?record_id=12585.

IOM found that family planning—"helping people have children when they want to and avoid conception when they do not—is a critical social and public health goal," and that the "federal government has a responsibility to support the attainment of this goal." IOM noted, for example, that family planning can prevent unintended and high-risk pregnancies, thereby reducing fetal, infant, and maternal mortality and morbidity. IOM also stated that the appropriate use of contraception can reduce abortion rates and cited "ample evidence that family planning services are cost-effective."[35]

IOM recommended that OFP develop and implement a multiyear evidence-based strategic plan.[36] IOM also made specific recommendations to improve program management and administration. For example, IOM recommended that

- program funding be increased so that statutory responsibilities can be met,
- methods of allocating funds be examined and improved,
- drug purchasing sources be consolidated,
- clinics' administrative burden be reduced,
- a single method be adopted for determining criteria for eligible services,
- transparency be increased,
- workforce needs be assessed, and
- program guidelines be evidence-based.[37]

Finally, IOM made recommendations to improve program evaluation. For example, IOM recommended that

- OFP collect additional data on client and system characteristics, the process and quality of care, and program outcomes;
- OFP fund and use a comprehensive framework for evaluating Title X;
- OFP obtain scientific input on its evaluation efforts; and
- evaluation findings be communicated to grantees, clinics, and others.[38]

In response to the IOM recommendations, OPA plans to have new Title X Family Planning Service Guidelines by the beginning of FY2013. These guidelines were developed over two years, during which expert panels reviewed the scientific literature. OPA states that the new guidelines will have "a foundation of empirical evidence and information supporting clinical practice."[39]

---

[35] IOM, *A Review of the HHS Family Planning Program: Mission, Management, and Measurement of Results*, pp. 4, 70.

[36] IOM, *A Review of the HHS Family Planning Program: Mission, Management, and Measurement of Results*, p. 98.

[37] IOM, *A Review of the HHS Family Planning Program: Mission, Management, and Measurement of Results*, pp. 140-143.

[38] IOM, *A Review of the HHS Family Planning Program: Mission, Management, and Measurement of Results*, pp. 166-170.

[39] HHS, HRSA, *Fiscal Year 2013 Justification of Estimates for Appropriations Committees*, p. 351.

Also in response to the IOM report, HHS has a contract with IOM to convene a Standing Committee to advise the Title X program. According to the FY2013 HRSA *Justification*, the Standing Committee is advising the program on the following areas related to report recommendations: strategic planning, workforce planning, improving data collection on program performance, and improving communication and transparency. The Standing Committee is also examining the roles of family planning, reproductive health, and Title X in health reform.[40]

The Patient Protection and Affordable Care Act and Title X

The Patient Protection and Affordable Care Act (ACA) has numerous provisions that may impact Title X clinics.[41] Notably, ACA increases access to health insurance.[42] (In 2010, 67% of Title X clients were uninsured.[43]) Federal ACA regulations and guidance will also require most health plans and health insurers to cover contraceptive services without cost-sharing.

ACA has several provisions that may increase health insurance coverage in the populations currently served by Title X. These provisions could help free up funds that Title X clinics currently spend on serving the uninsured. For example,

- States can expand Medicaid eligibility to include most nonelderly, nonpregnant individuals with income at or below 133% of FPL, effectively 138% FPL with the 5% income disregard.[44] (In 2010, 69% of Title X clients had incomes under 101% of FPL; another 15% had incomes between 101% and 150% of FPL.)[45]

---

[40] HHS, HRSA, *Fiscal Year 2013 Justification of Estimates for Appropriations Committees*, pp. 350-351. IOM, Standing Committee on Family Planning, http://www.iom.edu/Activities/Women/FamilyPlanning.aspx.

[41] The Patient Protection and Affordable Care Act (P.L. 111-148, March 23, 2010) was amended by the Health Care Education and Reconciliation Act of 2010 (P.L. 111-152, March 30, 2010). These acts will be collectively referred to in this report as "ACA."

[42] The Congressional Budget Office estimates that the share of nonelderly residents with insurance will grow from 80% in 2012 to 89% by 2022. Congressional Budget Office, *Estimates for the Insurance Coverage Provisions of the Affordable Care Act Updated for the Recent Supreme Court Decision*, July 24, 2012, p. 20, http://cbo.gov/publication/43472.

[43] Christina Fowler, Stacey Lloyd, Julia Gable, Jiantong Wang, and Kathleen Krieger, *Family Planning Annual Report: 2010 National Summary*, pp. 21, 23.

[44] P.L. 111-148, §2001 as modified by §10201; P.L. 111-152, §1004 and §1201. This provision is summarized in CRS Report R41210, *Medicaid and the State Children's Health Insurance Program (CHIP) Provisions in ACA: Summary and Timeline*, by Evelyne P. Baumrucker et al., and CRS Report RL33202, *Medicaid: A Primer*, by Elicia J. Herz. See also *To Be or Not to Be a "New Program"? What does NFIB v. Sebelius Mean for Implementation of the Affordable Care Act's Medicaid Expansion Provision?*, by Kathleen Swendiman, http://www.crs.gov/analysis/legalsidebar/pages/details.aspx?ProdId=121. All state Medicaid programs are mandated to include family planning services and supplies in their benefit packages, with no cost-sharing. For those in the new eligibility group, states receive a federal matching rate of 100% in 2014 through 2016, including for family planning expenditures, gradually declining to 90% in 2020 and thereafter. For all other Medicaid enrollees, states receive an enhanced federal matching rate of 90% for family planning expenditures.

[45] Christina Fowler, Stacey Lloyd, Julia Gable, Jiantong Wang, and Kathleen Krieger, *Family Planning Annual Report: 2010 National Summary*, p. 22.

- ACA gave states the option, through a Medicaid state plan amendment, of providing targeted Medicaid family planning services and supplies to certain individuals who would otherwise be ineligible for Medicaid.[46]

- ACA requires most private health plans that cover dependents to continue to make such coverage available for young adult children under the age of 26.[47] (In 2010, 53% of Title X clients were younger than 25 years old; another 21% were aged 25 to 29.)[48]

- Beginning in 2014, ACA will provide certain individuals and small businesses with access to private health plans through new health insurance exchanges and will subsidize the premium costs for certain individuals.[49]

- Beginning in 2014, ACA's individual mandate provision will require most individuals to have health insurance or pay a penalty.[50]

ACA provisions to expand health insurance coverage are described in CRS Report R41664, *ACA: A Brief Overview of the Law, Implementation, and Legal Challenges*, coordinated by C. Stephen Redhead.

OPA has established FY2012 Program Priorities to guide the project plans of family planning services grantees. In response to ACA, among the priorities is improving Title X clinics' ability to bill Medicaid and private health insurance:

> Identifying specific strategies for addressing the provisions of health care reform ("The Patient Protection and Affordable Care Act"), and for adapting delivery of family planning and reproductive health services to a changing health care environment, and assisting clients with navigating the changing health care system. This includes, but is not limited to, enhancing the ability of Title X clinics to bill third party payers, private insurance, and Medicaid.[51]

---

[46] P.L. 111-148, §2303. This provision was effective upon enactment. Prior to ACA, states could provide these Medicaid family planning expansions only by obtaining special waivers. This provision is summarized in CRS Report R41210, *Medicaid and the State Children's Health Insurance Program (CHIP) Provisions in ACA: Summary and Timeline*, by Evelyne P. Baumrucker et al. As of August 1, 2012, eight states have had state plan amendments approved under this new authority. Guttmacher Institute, State Policies in Brief as of August 1, 2012: Medicaid Family Planning Eligibility Expansion, http://www.guttmacher.org/statecenter/spibs/spib_SMFPE.pdf. Federal guidance is provided in Cindy Mann, Director, Center for Medicaid, CHIP and Survey & Certification, *State Medicaid Directors Letter #10-013, Family Planning Services Option and New Benefit Rules for Benchmark Plans*, July 2, 2010, https://www.cms.gov/smdl/downloads/SMD10013.pdf.

[47] P.L. 111-148, §1001, as amended by P.L. 111-152, §2301. This dependent coverage provision is effective for plan years beginning on or after September 23, 2010. The provision is summarized in CRS Report R41220, *Preexisting Condition Exclusion Provisions for Children and Dependent Coverage under the Patient Protection and Affordable Care Act (ACA)*, by Bernadette Fernandez.

[48] Christina Fowler, Stacey Lloyd, Julia Gable, Jiantong Wang, and Kathleen Krieger, *Family Planning Annual Report: 2010 National Summary*, p. 11.

[49] To ensure access for low-income individuals, most exchange plans will be required to have a sufficient number and geographic distribution of "essential community providers," which include Title X projects. HHS, "Patient Protection and Affordable Care Act; Establishment of Exchanges and Qualified Health Plans; Exchange Standards for Employers," 77 *Federal Register* 18470, March 27, 2012; 45 C.F.R. § 156.235.

[50] P.L. 111-148, §1501 and §10106, as amended by P.L. 111-152, §1002. This provision is summarized in CRS Report R41331, *Individual Mandate and Related Information Requirements under ACA*, by Janemarie Mulvey and Hinda Chaikind.

[51] HHS, OPA, *Title X Family Planning Program Priorities*, http://www.hhs.gov/opa/title-x-family-planning/title-x- (continued...)

Title X clinics could also provide enrollment assistance to clients who become newly eligible for Medicaid or exchange plans.[52] Title X supporters state that, although clinics currently funded by Title X could see increased revenues from Medicaid and private insurance after 2014, the Title X program will still be necessary:

> In addition to medical care, Title X supports activities that are not reimbursable under Medicaid and commercial insurance plans... Title X has made a major contribution to the training of clinicians; that need remains today... Title X helps to support staff salaries, not just for clinicians but for front-desk staff, educators and finance and administrative staff. Title X provides for individual patient education as well as community-level outreach and public education about family planning and women's health issues. Title X also helps to support the infrastructure necessary to keep the doors open—subsidizing rent, utilities and infrastructure needs like health information technology.[53]

Some advocates note that even after 2014, family planning services will still be sought by uninsured persons and dependents who, for confidentiality reasons, might not wish to bill reproductive health services to their parent's or spouse's health insurance.[54] Advocates maintain that even after 2014, there will still be strong demand for safety net providers, such as many Title X clinics, that provide health care to underserved populations.[55]

ACA requires most private health plans to cover certain preventive services for women without cost-sharing.[56] HHS commissioned IOM to recommend preventive services to be included in this requirement.[57] Adopting the IOM recommendations, federal rules and guidelines require that most health plans cover, without cost-sharing, "All Food and Drug Administration approved contraceptive methods, sterilization procedures, and patient education and counseling for all women with reproductive capacity," as prescribed.[58] Some have noted that this requirement, by

---

(...continued)

policies/program-priorities/.

[52] Adam Sonfield, "Implementing the Affordable Care Act: Enrollment Strategies and the U.S. Family Planning Effort," *Guttmacher Policy Review*, vol. 14, no. 4 (fall 2011), pp. 20-25. Rachel Benson Gold, "The Role of Family Planning Centers as Gateways To Health Coverage and Care ," *Guttmacher Policy Review*, vol. 14, no. 2 (spring 2011), pp. 15-19.

[53] Clare Coleman and Kirtly Parker Jones, "Title X: A Proud Past, An Uncertain Future," *Contraception*, vol. 84 (September 2011), pp. 209-211, http://www.arhp.org/publications-and-resources/contraception-journal/september-2011.

[54] The Congressional Budget Office estimates that about 30 million nonelderly residents will remain uninsured in 2022. Congressional Budget Office, *Estimates for the Insurance Coverage Provisions of the Affordable Care Act Updated for the Recent Supreme Court Decision*, July 24, 2012, p. 20. Confidentiality issues are discussed in Rachel Benson Gold, "Unintended Consequences: How Insurance Processes Inadvertently Abrogate Patient Confidentiality," *Guttmacher Policy Review*, vol. 12, no. 4 (fall 2009), pp. 12-16, http://www.guttmacher.org/pubs/gpr/12/4/gpr120412.html.

[55] Leighton Ku, Emily Jones, and Peter Shin et al., "Safety-Net Providers After Health Care Reform: Lessons from Massachusetts," *Archives of Internal Medicine*, vol. 171, no. 15 (August 2011), pp. 1379-1384. Massachusetts passed its health reform law in 2006. The authors found that between 2005 and 2009, the state's community health centers (which include some Title X clinics) saw a 31% increase in number of clients served. OPA's *Family Planning Annual Reports* indicate that between 2005 and 2010, the number of Title X clients in Massachusetts declined 7%, from 73,784 in 2005 to 68,446 in 2010. Nationally over the same time period, the number of Title X clients increased 4%, from 5.003 million in 2005 to 5.225 million in 2010. HHS, OPA, *Family Planning Annual Reports,* http://www.hhs.gov/opa/title-x-family-planning/research-and-data/fp-annual-reports/#fpar.

[56] P.L. 111-148, §1101.

[57] IOM, *Clinical Preventive Services for Women: Closing the Gaps* (Washington, DC: The National Academies Press, 2011), http://www.nap.edu/catalog.php?record_id=13181.

[58] The requirement is effective for plan years beginning on or after August 1, 2012, with some exceptions for religious (continued...)

removing up-front cost barriers, could result in more women switching to longer-acting contraceptive methods, such as hormonal implants and intrauterine devices.[59] The HRSA *Justification* notes that in FY2013, "Family planning centers will be encouraged and trained to provide a broad range of contraceptives, with a focus on expanding the availability of long-acting reversible methods."[60]

ACA may also impact Title X clinics in other ways. For example, because ACA increased the rebate percentage drug makers pay on drugs purchased for Medicaid beneficiaries, Title X clinics likely will receive larger discounts on drugs obtained through the 340B drug discount program.[61] ACA also increases funding for teen pregnancy prevention efforts, expands healthcare workforce programs, and increases funding for community health centers.[62] HHS has a contract with IOM to convene a Standing Committee to advise the Title X program. Among other topics, the IOM Standing Committee is examining the roles of family planning, reproductive health, and Title X in health reform.[63]

Abortion and Title X

The law prohibits the use of Title X funds in programs where abortion is a method of family planning.[64] On July 3, 2000, OPA released a final rule with respect to abortion services in family

---

(...continued)

entities. Condoms and vasectomies are not included. HHS, HRSA, *Women's Preventive Services: Required Health Plan Coverage Guidelines*, http://www.hrsa.gov/womensguidelines/. Health and Human Services Department, the Employee Benefits Security Administration, and the Internal Revenue Service, "Group Health Plans and Health Insurance Issuers Relating to Coverage of Preventive Services Under the Patient Protection and Affordable Care Act," 77 *Federal Register* 8725, February 15, 2012. Health and Human Services Department, the Employee Benefits Security Administration, and the Internal Revenue Service, "Certain Preventive Services Under the Affordable Care Act," 77 *Federal Register* 16502, Footnote 2, March 21, 2012. The rules and guidelines are discussed in CRS Report R42370, *Preventive Health Services Regulations: Religious Institutions' Objections to Contraceptive Coverage*, by Cynthia Brougher.

[59] Michelle Andrews, "Insurance Coverage Might Steer Women To Costlier—But More Effective—Birth Control," *Kaiser Health News*, February 20, 2012, http://www.kaiserhealthnews.org/Features/Insuring-Your-Health/2012/contraceptives-coverage-022112.aspx. Kelly Cleland, Jeffrey F. Peipert, and Carolyn Westhoff et al., "Family Planning as a Cost-Saving Preventive Health Service," *The New England Journal of Medicine*, vol. 364 (May 5, 2011), p. e37.

[60] HHS, HRSA, *Fiscal Year 2013 Justification of Estimates for Appropriations Committees*, p. 351.

[61] P.L. 111-148, §2501. Title X clinics are among the entities eligible to receive discounts on certain drugs' prices under Section 340B of the Public Health Service Act. The maximum prices that drug manufacturers can charge 340B entities are calculated using the Medicaid rebate formula. The ACA provision is summarized in CRS Report R41210, *Medicaid and the State Children's Health Insurance Program (CHIP) Provisions in ACA: Summary and Timeline*, by Evelyne P. Baumrucker et al. The 340B program website is http://www.hrsa.gov/opa. There were 3,868 Title X clinic sites enrolled in the 340B program as of July 1, 2011. U.S. Government Accountability Office, *Drug Pricing: Manufacturer Discounts in the 340B Program Offer Benefits, but Federal Oversight Needs Improvement*, GAO-11-836, September 23, 2011, p. 39, http://gao.gov/products/GAO-11-836.

[62] These and other ACA provisions that could potentially impact Title X clinics are summarized in CRS Report R41278, *Public Health, Workforce, Quality, and Related Provisions in PPACA: Summary and Timeline*, coordinated by C. Stephen Redhead and Erin D. Williams, and CRS Report R41210, *Medicaid and the State Children's Health Insurance Program (CHIP) Provisions in ACA: Summary and Timeline*, by Evelyne P. Baumrucker et al.

[63] IOM, *Standing Committee on Family Planning*, http://www.iom.edu/Activities/Women/FamilyPlanning.aspx. HHS, HRSA, *Fiscal Year 2013 Justification of Estimates for Appropriations Committees*, p. 351.

[64] 42 U.S.C. §300a-6. In addition, language in annual Departments of Labor, Health and Human Services, and Education, and Related Agencies Appropriations bills have also prohibited the use of Title X funds for abortions (in FY2012, this provision appeared in P.L. 112-74, 125 Stat. 1066). For background on abortion funding restrictions in (continued...)

planning projects.[65] The rule updated and revised regulations that had been in effect since 1988.[66] The major revision revoked the "gag rule," which restricted family planning grantees from providing abortion-related information. The regulation at 42 C.F.R. Section 59.5 had required, and continues to require, that abortion not be provided as a method of family planning. The July 3, 2000, rule amended the section to add the requirement that a project must give pregnant women the opportunity to receive information and counseling on each of the following options: prenatal care and delivery; infant care, foster care, or adoption; and pregnancy termination. If the woman requests such information and counseling, the project must give "neutral, factual information and nondirective counseling on each of the options, and referral upon request, except with respect to any option(s) about which the pregnant woman indicates she does not wish to receive such information and counseling."[67]

According to OPA, family planning projects that receive Title X funds are closely monitored to ensure that federal funds are used appropriately and that funds are not used for prohibited activities such as abortion. The prohibition on abortion does not apply to all the activities of a Title X grantee, but only to activities that are part of the Title X project. The grantee's abortion activities must be "separate and distinct" from the Title X project activities.[68] Safeguards to maintain this separation include (1) careful review of grant applications to ensure that the applicant understands the requirements and has the capacity to comply with all requirements; (2) independent financial audits to examine whether there is a system to account for program-funded activities and non-allowable program activities; (3) yearly comprehensive reviews of the grantees' financial status and budget report; and (4) periodic and comprehensive program reviews and site visits by OPA regional offices.[69]

It is unclear exactly how many Title X clinics also provide abortions through their non-Title X activities. In 2004, following appropriations conference report directions, HHS surveyed its Title X grantees on whether their clinic sites also provided abortions with non-federal funds.[70] Grantees were informed that responses were voluntary and "without consequence, or threat of consequence, to non-responsiveness." The survey did not request any identifying information. HHS mailed surveys to 86 grantees and received 46 responses. Of these, 9 indicated that at least one of their clinic sites (17 clinic sites in all) also provided abortions with non-federal funds, and

---

(...continued)

general, see CRS Report RL33467, *Abortion: Judicial History and Legislative Response*, by Jon O. Shimabukuro.

[65] HHS, OPA, "Standards of Compliance for Abortion-Related Services in Family Planning Services Projects," 65 *Federal Register* 41270-41280, July 3, 2000; and HHS, OPA, "Provision of Abortion-Related Services in Family Planning Services Projects, " 65 *Federal Register* 41281-41282, July 3, 2000.

[66] 42 C.F.R. Part 59, "Grants for family planning services."

[67] On December 19, 2008, HHS published a provider conscience rule which, according to HHS, is inconsistent with the requirement that Title X grantees provide clients with abortion referrals upon request. 73 *Federal Register* 78087. This is discussed below in "Provider Conscience Rule."

[68] 65 *Federal Register* 41281-41282, July 3, 2000.

[69] E-mail from Barbara Clark, HHS, Office of the Assistant Secretary for Legislation, August 24, 2006. See also *OPA Program Instruction Series, OPA 11-01: Title X Grantee Compliance with Grant Requirements and Applicable Federal and State Law, including State Reporting Laws*, Letter from Marilyn J. Keefe, Deputy Assistant Secretary for Population Affairs, to Regional Health Administrators, Regions I-X; Title X Grantees, March 1, 2011, http://www.hhs.gov/opa/pdf/opa-11-01-program-instruction-re-compliance.pdf.

[70] HHS, *Report to Congress Regarding the Number of Family Planning Sites Funded Under Title X of the Public Health Service Act That Also Provide Abortions with Non-Federal Funds*, 2004. HHS was directed to conduct the survey by FY2004 appropriations conference report H.Rept. 108-401, pp. 800-801.

34 indicated that none of their clinic sites provided abortions with non-federal funds; 3 responses had no numerical data or said the information was unknown.

Title X supporters argue that family planning reduces unintended pregnancies, thereby reducing abortion.[71] HHS estimates that Title X family planning services helped avert 996,000 unintended pregnancies in 2010.[72] The Guttmacher Institute estimates that clinics receiving Title X funds helped avert 406,200 abortions in 2008.[73]

On the other hand, Title X critics argue that federal funds should be withheld from any organization that performs or promotes abortions, such as the Planned Parenthood Federation of America. These critics argue that federal funding for non-abortion activities frees up Planned Parenthood's other resources for its abortion activities.[74] Some critics also argue that if a family planning program is operated by an organization that also performs abortions, the implicit assumption and the message to clients is that abortion is a method of family planning.[75]

Teenage Pregnancy and Title X

In 2010, 22% of Title X clients were aged 19 or younger.[76] Critics argue that by funding Title X, the federal government is implicitly sanctioning nonmarital sexual activity among teens. These critics argue that a reduced teenage pregnancy rate could be achieved if family planning programs emphasized efforts to convince teens to delay sexual activity, rather than efforts to decrease the percentage of sexually active teens who become pregnant.[77] (See CRS Report RS20301, *Teenage Pregnancy Prevention: Statistics and Programs*, by Carmen Solomon-Fears, for a broader discussion of teen pregnancy.)

---

[71] Examples of this argument can be found in Rachel Benson Gold, Adam Sonfield, and Cory L. Richards, et al., *Next Steps for America's Family Planning Program: Leveraging the Potential of Medicaid and Title X in an Evolving Health Care System*, Guttmacher Institute, New York, 2009, pp. 16-17, http://www.guttmacher.org/pubs/NextSteps.pdf, and in U.S. Congress, Senate Committee on Appropriations, Subcommittee on Labor, Health and Human Services, Education, and Related Agencies, *Threat to Title X and Other Women's Health Services*, 104th Cong., 1st sess., August 10, 1995, S.Hrg. 104-416 (Washington: GPO, 1996), pp. 16-21.

[72] HHS, HRSA, *Fiscal Year 2013 Justification of Estimates for Appropriations Committees*, p. 349.

[73] Jennifer J. Frost, Stanley K. Henshaw, and Adam Sonfeld, *Contraceptive needs and services: national and state data, 2008 update*, Guttmacher Institute, New York, NY, 2010, p. 16, http://www.guttmacher.org/pubs/win/contraceptive-needs-2008.pdf.

[74] Examples of this argument can be found in House debate, *Congressional Record*, daily edition, vol. 154, no. 112 (July 9, 2008), pp. H6320-H6326. In 2010, 329,445 abortion procedures were performed by Planned Parenthood affiliates, comprising 3% of Planned Parenthood services that year, according to the Planned Parenthood Federation of America, *Planned Parenthood Services Fact Sheet*, 2012, p. 2, http://www.plannedparenthood.org/files/PPFA/PP_Services.pdf.

[75] An example of these arguments can be found in U.S. Congress, Senate Committee on Appropriations, Subcommittee on Labor, Health and Human Services, Education, and Related Agencies, *Threat to Title X and Other Women's Health Services*, pp. 22-35.

[76] Christina Fowler, Stacey Lloyd, Julia Gable, Jiantong Wang, and Kathleen Krieger, *Family Planning Annual Report: 2010 National Summary*, p. 9.

[77] An example of these arguments can be found in U.S. Congress, Senate Committee on Appropriations, Subcommittee on Labor, Health and Human Services, Education, and Related Agencies, *Threat to Title X and Other Women's Health Services*, pp. 22-35.

The program's supporters, on the other hand, argue that the Title X program should be expanded to serve more people in order to reduce the rate of unintended pregnancies. According to HHS, in 2010, Title X family planning services helped avert an estimated 219,000 unintended teen pregnancies.[78] Supporters of expanding family planning services argue that the United States has a higher teen pregnancy rate than some countries (such as Sweden) where a similar percentage of teens are sexually active, in part because U.S. teens use contraception less consistently.[79]

Confidentiality for Minors and Title X

Confidentiality is required for personal information about Title X services provided to individuals.[80] Regarding services to minors, Title X project guidelines state:

> Adolescents must be assured that the counseling sessions are confidential and, if follow-up is necessary, every attempt will be made to assure the privacy of the individual. However, counselors should encourage family participation in the decision of minors to seek family planning services and provide counseling to minors on resisting attempts to coerce minors into engaging in sexual activities. Title X projects may not require written consent of parents or guardians for the provision of services to minors. Nor can the project notify parents or guardians before or after a minor has requested and received Title X family planning services.[81]

Although minors are to receive confidential services, Title X providers are not exempt from state notification and reporting laws on child abuse, child molestation, sexual abuse, rape, or incest.[82]

As for payment of services provided to minors, Title X regulations indicate that "unemancipated minors who wish to receive services on a confidential basis must be considered on the basis of

---

[78] HHS, HRSA, *Fiscal Year 2013 Justification of Estimates for Appropriations Committees*, p. 349. See also the discussion of publicly funded family planning services in "Programs to Reduce Unintended Pregnancy," in The Institute of Medicine, *The Best Intentions: Unintended Pregnancy and the Well-Being of Children and Families* (Washington: National Academy Press, 1995), p. 220, http://www.nap.edu/catalog.php?record_id=4903.

[79] An example of these arguments can be found in U.S. Congress, Senate Committee on Appropriations, Subcommittee on Labor, Health and Human Services, Education, and Related Agencies, *Threat to Title X and Other Women's Health Services*, pp. 16-21. See also Jacqueline E. Darroch, et al., "Differences in Teenage Pregnancy Rates Among Five Developed Countries: The Roles of Sexual Activity and Contraceptive Use," *Family Planning Perspectives*, vol. 33, no. 6 (November/December 2001), pp. 244-251.

[80] 42 C.F.R. §59.11. Also, several court cases have interpreted Title X statute as supporting confidentiality for minors; see Glenn A. Guarino, "Provision of family planning services under Title X of Public Health Service Act (42 U.S.C.A. §300-300a-8) and implementing regulations," *American Law Reports Federal*, 1985, 71 A.L.R. Fed. 961.

[81] HHS, Office of Family Planning, *Program Guidelines For Project Grants For Family Planning Services*, January 2001, p. 25, http://www.hhs.gov/opa/title-x-family-planning/title-x-policies/program-guidelines/. For an overview of Title X efforts to encourage family participation, see RTI International, *An Assessment of Parent Involvement Strategies in Programs Serving Adolescents: Final Report*, 2007, http://www.hhs.gov/opa/pdfs/parent-involvement-final-report.pdf. The report found that parent involvement is associated with several positive outcomes, such as delayed sexual initiation and lower rates of pregnancy and sexually transmitted infections.

[82] P.L. 112-74, Division F, Departments of Labor, Health and Human Services, and Education, and Related Agencies Appropriations Act, 2010, Title II, Department of Health and Human Services, §210, 125 Stat. 1083. *OPA Program Instruction Series, OPA 11-01: Title X Grantee Compliance with Grant Requirements and Applicable Federal and State Law, including State Reporting Laws*, Letter from Marilyn J. Keefe, Deputy Assistant Secretary for Population Affairs, to Regional Health Administrators, Regions I-X; Title X Grantees, March 1, 2011, http://www.hhs.gov/opa/pdf/opa-11-01-program-instruction-re-compliance.pdf.

their own resources."[83] The project guidelines instruct that "Eligibility for discounts for minors who receive confidential services must be based on the income of the minor."[84]

Supporters of confidentiality argue that parental notification or parental consent requirements would lead some sexually active adolescents to delay or forgo family planning services, thereby increasing their risk of pregnancy or sexually transmitted diseases.[85]

Critics argue that confidentiality requirements can interfere with parents' right to know of and to guide their children's health care. Some critics also disagree with discounts for minors without regard to parents' income, because the Title X program was intended to serve "low-income families."[86]

Planned Parenthood and Title X

The Planned Parenthood Federation of America (PPFA) operates through a national office and 77 affiliates, which operate nearly 800 local health centers.[87] Affiliates participating in Title X can receive funds directly from HHS or indirectly from other Title X grantees, such as their state or local health departments. PPFA and its affiliates receive about $66 million in annual Title X funding, according to the PPFA Washington Office.[88]

In May 2010, the Government Accountability Office (GAO) released a report with data on the obligations and expenditures of federal funds for several nonprofit organizations, including PPFA and its affiliates.[89]

According to the GAO report, in FY2009, HHS reported obligating to Planned Parenthood and its affiliates $18.2 million through the Title X Family Planning Services program and $0.3 million through Title X Family Planning Service Delivery Improvement Research Grants.[90] These figures reflect funds that HHS provided directly to these organizations. They do not include Title X funds

---

[83] 42 C.F.R. §59.2.

[84] HHS, Office of Family Planning, *Program Guidelines For Project Grants For Family Planning Services*, January 2001, p. 8.

[85] An example of this argument is in Rachel K. Jones, Alison Purcell, and Susheela Singh et al., "Adolescents' Reports of Parental Knowledge of Adolescents' Use of Sexual Health Services and Their Reactions to Mandated Parental Notification for Prescription Contraception," *JAMA*, vol. 293, no. 3 (January 19, 2005), pp. 340-348. See also the staff quotations in RTI International, *An Assessment of Parent Involvement Strategies in Programs Serving Adolescents: Final Report*, 2007, pp. 5-10.

[86] Examples of these arguments appear in *Congressional Record*, daily edition, vol. 142 (July 11, 1996), pp. H7348-H 7349, and U.S. Congress, Senate Committee on Appropriations, Subcommittee on Labor, Health and Human Services, Education, and Related Agencies, *Threat to Title X and Other Women's Health Services*, 104th Cong., 1st sess., August 10, 1995, S.Hrg. 104-416 (Washington: GPO, 1996), pp. 22-23. See also the discussion in RTI International, *An Assessment of Parent Involvement Strategies in Programs Serving Adolescents: Final Report*, 2007, pp. 5-9.

[87] Planned Parenthood Federation of America, *Planned Parenthood at a Glance*, http://www.plannedparenthood.org/about-us/who-we-are/planned-parenthood-glance-5552.htm.

[88] E-mail from Ellen Weissfeld, Public Policy Coordinator, Planned Parenthood Federation of America, April 12, 2011.

[89] U.S. Government Accountability Office (GAO), *Federal Funds: Fiscal Years 2002-2009 Obligations, Disbursements, and Expenditures for Selected Organizations Involved in Health-Related Activities*, GAO-10-533R, May 28, 2010, http://www.gao.gov/products/GAO-10-533R.

[90] GAO, *Federal Funds: Fiscal Years 2002-2009 Obligations, Disbursements, and Expenditures for Selected Organizations Involved in Health-Related Activities*, p. 16.

that reached Planned Parenthood or its affiliates indirectly through subgrants or that passed through from state agencies or other organizations.

The GAO report also showed Planned Parenthood's expenditures of Title X funds. These expenditures were identified through audit reports that Planned Parenthood and its affiliates submitted to comply with Office of Management and Budget (OMB) audit requirements.[91] Expenditures include federal funds provided directly or indirectly to these organizations. The most recent expenditure data were from FY2008, when Planned Parenthood and its affiliates reported spending $53 million from the Title X Family Planning Services program.[92]

Provider Conscience Rule

Overview

Several already existing federal restrictions protect health care providers from being coerced to provide certain services to which they object. These statutory restrictions prohibit recipients of certain federal funds from discriminating against such providers. These restrictions include the Church Amendment (which protects those with religious or moral objections to abortion and sterilization), Public Health Service (PHS) Act Section 245 (which protects certain individuals, medical schools, and training programs that will not provide, perform, make arrangements for, or refer for abortions or abortion training), and the Weldon Amendment (which protects certain entities that will not provide, pay for, provide coverage for, or refer for abortions).[93]

In the December 19, 2008, *Federal Register*, HHS published a final rule, often called the provider conscience rule, that was intended to increase awareness of these existing restrictions.[94] Some critics argued that the rule would limit patients' access to contraception, and that it conflicted with the Title X requirement that grantees provide pregnant women, upon request, nondirective counseling and referrals on several options including abortion.

The rule became effective January 20, 2009. In the March 10, 2009, *Federal Register*, HHS proposed to rescind the provider conscience rule and invited public comments.[95]

---

[91] Organizations with annual expenditures of federal funds of $500,000 or more are required to have an audit. The GAO report includes expenditure data from 85 Planned Parenthood affiliates. GAO, *Federal Funds: Fiscal Years 2002-2009 Obligations, Disbursements, and Expenditures for Selected Organizations Involved in Health-Related Activities*, p. 10 footnote b, p. 22 footnote 1.

[92] GAO, *Federal Funds: Fiscal Years 2002-2009 Obligations, Disbursements, and Expenditures for Selected Organizations Involved in Health-Related Activities*, p. 25.

[93] More background about these and other federal provider conscience provisions is in CRS Report R40722, *Health Care Providers' Religious Objections to Medical Treatment: Legal Issues Related to Religious Discrimination in Employment and Conscience Clause Provisions*, by Cynthia Brougher and Edward C. Liu, and CRS Report RL34703, *The History and Effect of Abortion Conscience Clause Laws*, by Jon O. Shimabukuro. See also HHS, Office for Civil Rights (OCR), *Overview of Federal Statutory Health Care Provider Conscience Protections*, http://www.hhs.gov/ocr/civilrights/faq/providerconsciencefaq.html, and *Federal Health Care Conscience Protection Statutes*, http://www.hhs.gov/ocr/civilrights/understanding/ConscienceProtect/index.html.

[94] U.S. Department of Health and Human Services, "Ensuring Department of Health and Human Services Funds Do Not Support Coercive or Discriminatory Policies or Practices in Violation of Federal Law," 73 *Federal Register* 78072–78101, December 19, 2008, http://federalregister.gov/a/E8-30134.

[95] HHS, "Rescission of the Regulation Entitled 'Ensuring That Department of Health and Human Services Funds Do (continued...)

Title X (Public Health Service Act) Family Planning Program

In the February 23, 2011, *Federal Register*, HHS rescinded most of the rule, except for a provision that the HHS Office for Civil Rights will handle complaints based on federal health care provider conscience protection restrictions. HHS stated that parts of the 2008 rule were "unclear and potentially overbroad in scope," and noted that the rescission "does not alter or affect the federal statutory health care provider conscience protections" that already exist.[96]

2008 Rule

The 2008 provider conscience rule stated that entities carrying out HHS health service programs shall not require individuals "to perform or assist in the performance of any part of a health service program or research activity funded by the Department if such service or activity would be contrary to his religious beliefs or moral convictions."[97] The rule defined *assist in the performance* as participating in any activity with a "reasonable connection" to the objectionable procedure or health service, including "counseling, referral, training, and other arrangements" for the procedure or health service.[98]

The rule prohibited recipients of HHS appropriations act funds from subjecting institutions or individuals to discrimination because they did not refer patients for abortions.[99] Also, the rule prohibited recipients of grants under the Public Health Service Act from discriminating against physicians or other health care professionals because they refused to assist in the performance of sterilization or abortion based on religious beliefs or moral convictions.[100]

Before publishing the final rule, HHS solicited public comments.[101] Some commenters argued that the rule was inconsistent with the Title X regulatory requirement that grantees provide pregnant women, upon request, nondirective counseling and referrals on several options including abortion.[102] The Title X requirement states that if the woman requests such information and counseling, the project must give "neutral, factual information and nondirective counseling on each of the options, and referral upon request, except with respect to any option(s) about which the pregnant woman indicates she does not wish to receive such information and counseling."[103]

(...continued)
Not Support Coercive or Discriminatory Support Coercive or Discriminatory Federal Law'; Proposal," 74 *Federal Register* 10207-10211, March 10, 2009, http://federalregister.gov/a/E9-5067. Many of the public comments are posted at http://www.regulations.gov/#!docketDetail;D=HHS-OPHS-2009-0001.

[96] HHS, "Regulation for the Enforcement of Federal Health Care Provider Conscience Protection Laws," 76 *Federal Register* 9969, February 23, 2011, http://federalregister.gov/a/2011-3993.

[97] 73 *Federal Register* 79097, 79098, §88.3(g)(1), §88.4(d)(1).

[98] 73 *Federal Register* 78097, §88.2.

[99] 73 *Federal Register* 78097, 78098, §88.3(c), §88.4(b)(2).

[100] 73 *Federal Register* 78097, 78098, §88.3(f)(1), §88.4(c)(1).

[101] Comments may be viewed at http://www.regulations.gov/#!docketDetail;D=HHS-OS-2008-0011. (Check the "Public Submissions" box).

[102] Examples of such comments include Letter from Sharon L. Camp, President and CEO, Guttmacher Institute, to HHS, September 24, 2008, http://www.guttmacher.org/media/resources/2008/09/24/GuttmacherInstitute-re-ConscienceRegulation.pdf, and Letter from Caroline Fredrickson, Director, Washington Legislative Office, American Civil Liberties Union (ACLU), Louise Melling, Director, Reproductive Freedom Project, ACLU, and Vania Leveille, Washington Legislative Office, ACLU et al. to HHS, September 25, 2008, http://www.aclu.org/images/asset_upload_file467_36942.pdf.

[103] 42 C.F.R. §59(a)(5).

HHS responded that the provider conscience requirement did indeed conflict with the Title X requirement, so that in certain situations, OPA would not enforce the Title X referral regulation:

> With regards to the Title X program, Commenters are correct that the current regulatory requirement that grantees must provide counseling and referrals for abortion upon request (42 C.F.R. 59.5(a)(5)) is inconsistent with the health care provider conscience protection statutory provisions and this regulation. The Office of Population Affairs, which administers the Title X program, is aware of this conflict with the statutory requirements and, as such, would not enforce this Title X regulatory requirement on objecting grantees or applicants.[104]

The 2008 rule did not define the term *abortion*. Some commenters argued that by not defining abortion as excluding contraception, the rule could jeopardize Title X programs. HHS responded that "questions over the nature of abortion and the ending of a life are highly controversial and strongly debated," and so declined to issue a formal definition. HHS added that "nothing in this rule alters the obligation of federal Title X programs to deliver contraceptive services to clients in need as authorized by law and regulation."[105]

Some commenters argued that the rule would make it difficult for Title X clinics to screen job applicants to ensure that staff were willing to provide contraceptive services. HHS responded that job applicants would be unlikely to apply for, or be best qualified for, jobs where they object to the majority of the work. HHS explained further:

> To the extent a health care employer's adverse decision is based on an applicant's inability to perform the essential functions of a job, the decision would not typically constitute discrimination under the regulation even if the applicant had expressed an unwillingness to perform those functions on conscience grounds. However, an adverse decision predicated on an applicant's alleged "inability" could constitute unlawful discrimination if the employer's stated reasons are pretextual; for example, if the employer is using the definition of essential functions as a pretext for excluding applicants with certain religious beliefs or moral convictions.[106]

In response to comments that the rule would restrict patients' access to contraception, HHS responded that "we have found no evidence that these regulations will create new barriers in accessing contraception unless those contraceptives are currently delivered over the religious or moral objections of the provider."[107]

2011 Rule Rescission

In the February 23, 2011, *Federal Register*, HHS rescinded most of the 2008 final rule, except for a provision that the HHS Office for Civil Rights (OCR) will coordinate the handling of complaints based on federal provider conscience statutory restrictions.[108] HHS stated that "No

---

[104] 73 *Federal Register* 78087.

[105] 73 *Federal Register* 78077.

[106] 73 *Federal Register* 78084-78085.

[107] 73 *Federal Register* 78071-78072.

[108] HHS explained that the enforcement of statutory provider conscience protections would include "normal program compliance mechanisms." For example, HHS is expected to help violating entities come into compliance, and if entities still fail to comply, HHS "will consider all legal options," such as the termination of funds and the return of funds paid out in violation of the conscience statutes. HHS also stated that it is starting an initiative to increase awareness of (continued...)

regulations were required or necessary for the conscience protections contained in the Church Amendments, PHS Act, Section 245, and the Weldon Amendment to take effect," and that the rule rescission does not affect existing provider conscience statutory restrictions.[109]

As discussed above in "2008 Rule," some commenters had raised concerns about possible conflicts between the 2008 Rule and requirements governing certain HHS programs, including Title X. In the 2011 rule rescission, HHS stated that such conflicts would be addressed on a case-by-case basis:

> Health care entities must continue to comply with the long-established requirements of the statutes above governing Departmental programs. These statutes strike a careful balance between the rights of patients to access needed health care, and the conscience rights of health care providers. The conscience laws and the other federal statutes have operated side by side often for many decades. As repeals by implication are disfavored and laws are meant to be read in harmony, the Department fully intends to continue to enforce all the laws it has been charged with administering. The Department is partially rescinding the 2008 final rule in an attempt to address ambiguities that may have been caused in this area. The approach of a case by case investigation and, if necessary, enforcement will best enable the Department to deal with any perceived conflicts within concrete situations.[110]

As discussed in "2008 Rule," some commenters had raised concerns that the 2008 rule did not define "abortion" as excluding contraception. In rescinding the rule, HHS stated that "The provision of contraceptive services has never been defined as abortion in federal statute. There is no indication that the federal health care provider conscience statutes intended that the term 'abortion' included contraception."[111]

As discussed in "2008 Rule," some commenters had raised concerns that the 2008 rule could restrict some patients' access to contraception. HHS stated that it rescinded the rule in part because it "had the potential to negatively impact patient access to contraception and certain other medical services without a basis in federal conscience protection statutes." HHS reiterated that entities should continue to comply with their Title X obligations.[112]

(...continued)

federal provider conscience protections among grantees and health care providers. OCR includes provider conscience information in its education and outreach efforts and on its website, and HHS is amending its grant documents to clarify that recipients must comply with federal conscience protection laws. HHS, "Regulation for the Enforcement of Federal Health Care Provider Conscience Protection Laws," 76 *Federal Register* 9972, February 23, 2010.

[109] 76 *Federal Register* 9969, 9970.

[110] 76 *Federal Register* 9973.

[111] 76 *Federal Register* 9973.

[112] 76 *Federal Register* 9974.

Legislation in the 112th Congress

Several bills on the Title X program have been introduced in the 112th Congress.

Abortion Restrictions

H.R. 217, the Title X Abortion Provider Prohibition Act, was introduced January 7, 2011. The bill would prohibit Title X assistance to any entity unless it certifies that it will not perform, nor provide funds to any other entity that performs, an abortion during the period of assistance. The prohibition would not apply to hospitals, unless the hospital provides funds to a non-hospital entity that performs an abortion. The bill has exceptions for abortions performed in cases of rape, incest against a minor, or certain physician-certified cases where the woman is "in danger of death unless an abortion is performed." H.R. 217 would also require the HHS Secretary to provide Congress an annual report listing, for each entity receiving a Title X grant: information on any abortions it performed, the date that it last certified that it would not perform abortions, and any other entities to which it makes available funds received through Title X grants. The bill was referred to the House Committee on Energy and Commerce.

S. 96, the Title X Family Planning Act, was introduced January 25, 2011. It would prohibit Title X funds from going to entities that perform abortions or whose subgrantees perform abortions, except in certain physician-certified cases where the woman is "in danger of death unless an abortion is performed." This prohibition would not apply to hospitals, unless the hospital subgrants to a non-hospital entity that performs abortions. S. 96 would require Title X grant applicants to certify that they and their subgrantees adhere to the abortion prohibition. It would also require the HHS to provide Congress with an annual list of Title X grantees that perform abortions; if an entity appears on the list, it would be ineligible for subsequent fiscal year Title X funds unless it certifies that it no longer performs abortions. S. 96 was referred to the Senate Committee on Health, Education, Labor, and Pensions.

Other bills related to abortion are discussed in CRS Report RL33467, *Abortion: Judicial History and Legislative Response*, by Jon O. Shimabukuro.

Elimination of Title X Funds

H.R. 1, the Full-Year Continuing Appropriations Act, 2011, passed the House on February 19, 2011, and failed to pass the Senate on March 9, 2011. It would have eliminated funding for Title X for the remainder of FY2011. During House debate on H.R. 1, three amendments were submitted that would have struck the language eliminating funds for Title X.[113] One of those amendments would have also maintained FY2011 Title X funding at the FY2010 level of $317.491 million.[114] These amendments did not see floor action. During Senate debate on H.R. 1, S.Amdt. 149 was defeated; it was a substitute amendment that would have continued funding Title X for the remainder of FY2011 at the same rate of operations and under the same conditions as in FY2010. On April 15, 2011, P.L. 112-10, the Department of Defense and Full-Year

---

[113] Amendment no. 335, House amendments, *Congressional Record*, daily edition, February 14, 2011, p. H794; Amendment no. 386, House amendments, *Congressional Record*, daily edition, February 14, 2011, p. H796; Amendment no. 505, House amendments, *Congressional Record*, daily edition, February 15, 2011, p. H929.

[114] Amendment no. 335, House amendments, *Congressional Record*, daily edition, February 14, 2011, p. H794.

Continuing Appropriations Act, 2011, became law; it provided $299.400 million for Title X in FY2011.[115]

H.R. 408, the Spending Reduction Act of 2011, was introduced January 24, 2011. It would eliminate the Title X program, stating that "No funds appropriated or otherwise available to any Federal department or agency may be obligated or expended for" a list of programs including Title X. It was referred to the House Committees on Oversight and Government Reform, Natural Resources, Transportation and Infrastructure, Budget, Rules, Appropriations, Agriculture, Administration, Education and the Workforce, Energy and Commerce, Ways and Means, Financial Services, Judiciary, and Science, Space, and Technology.

S. 178, the Spending Reduction Act of 2011, was introduced January 25, 2011. It would eliminate the Title X program, stating that "No funds appropriated or otherwise available to any Federal department or agency may be obligated or expended for" a list of programs including Title X. It was referred to the Senate Committee on Finance.

H.R. 1099, the Taxpayers' Freedom of Conscience Act of 2011, was introduced March 15, 2011. It would prohibit federal officials from expending federal funds for "any population control or population planning program or any family planning activity (including any abortion procedure), irrespective of whether such program or activity is foreign or domestic." H.R. 1099 was referred to the House Committees on Foreign Affairs and Energy and Commerce.

H.R. 3070, the Departments of Labor, Health and Human Services, and Education, and Related Agencies Appropriations Act, 2012, was introduced September 29, 2011. The act's funds would be prohibited from being used to carry out Title X of the Public Health Service Act. H.R. 3070 was referred to the House Committee on Appropriations.

On July 18, 2012, the House Appropriations Subcommittee on Labor, Health and Human Services, Education, and Related Agencies approved a draft FY2013 Labor-HHS-Education bill.[116] The bill's funds would be prohibited from being used to carry out Title X of the Public Health Service Act.

Public Disclosure of Audits

S. 814, the Title X Transparency and Verification Act, was introduced April 13, 2011. It would require disclosure on the HHS website of the results of any audits conducted under Title X on any entity receiving Title X funds. S. 814 was referred to the Senate Committee on Health, Education, Labor, and Pensions.

---

[115] Section 1810 provides $300 million for Title X in FY2011. Section 1119 rescinds 0.2% across-the-board from most non-defense items including Title X.

[116] U.S. Congress, House Committee on Appropriations, Subcommittee on Labor, Health and Human Services, Education, and Related Agencies, *Making appropriations for the Departments of Labor, Health and Human Services, and Education, and related agencies for the fiscal year ending September 30, 2012, and for other purposes*, Draft bill, 112th Cong., 2nd sess., July 15, 2012, Sec. 219, p. 85, http://appropriations.house.gov/uploadedfiles/bills-112hr-sc-ap-fy13-laborhhsed.pdf.

Nondiscrimination on the Basis of Abortion Provision with Non-Title X Funds

H.R. 5650, the Protecting Women's Access to Health Care Act, was introduced May 9, 2012. It would prohibit Title X grantees and contractors from discriminating against a health care entity on the basis of whether it separately provides or refers for abortions, provides employees coverage of abortions, or provides or requires training in performing abortions. H.R. 5650 was referred to the House Committee on Energy and Commerce.

Limits on Means-Tested Welfare Spending

H.R. 1135, H.R. 1167, and S. 1904, all titled the Welfare Reform Act of 2011, would define "means-tested welfare spending" programs to include family planning, as well as more than 70 other federal programs. The bills would require a limit on aggregate means-tested welfare spending, no greater than the FY2007 level, adjusted for inflation. The limit would be enforced through the congressional budget process. Under H.R. 1135 and H.R. 1167, this limit would become effective "after any monthly rate of unemployment during the immediately preceding fiscal year is below 6.5 percent." Under S. 1904, this limit would become effective in FY2015 or "after any monthly rate of unemployment during the immediately preceding fiscal year is below 7.5%," whichever is earlier. Among other provisions, the bills would also require the President's Budget to provide information on total means-tested welfare spending. H.R. 1135 was introduced March 16, 2011, and referred to the House Committees on Ways and Means, Agriculture, the Budget, Rules, and Energy and Commerce. H.R. 1167 was introduced March 17, 2011, and referred to the same committees. S. 1904 was introduced November 17, 2011, and referred to the Senate Committee on Finance.

Restrictions on Funding to Planned Parenthood

H.Con.Res. 36 would have directed the House Clerk to make a correction in the enrollment of H.R. 1473, the Department of Defense and Full-Year Continuing Appropriations Act, 2011.[117] It would have prohibited funds under H.R. 1473 from being made available "for any purpose" to the Planned Parenthood Federation of America or any of its affiliates. On April 14, 2011, H.Con.Res. 36 passed the House and was defeated in the Senate.

H.Amdt. 95 to H.R. 1, the Full-Year Continuing Appropriations Act, 2011, would have prohibited the bill's funds from being made available "for any purpose" to PPFA or to any of 102 affiliates and offices listed in the amendment.[118] The House agreed to the amendment on February 18, 2011. H.R. 1 passed the House on February 19, 2011, and failed to pass the Senate on March 9, 2011. During Senate debate on H.R. 1, S.Amdt. 149 was defeated; it was a substitute amendment that did not mention Planned Parenthood and that would not have eliminated funds for Planned Parenthood. On April 15, 2011, P.L. 112-10, the Department of Defense and Full-Year Continuing Appropriations Act, 2011, became law; it did not mention Planned Parenthood and did not eliminate funds for Planned Parenthood.

---

[117] H.R. 1473 became P.L. 112-10 on April 15, 2011.

[118] Amendment no. 11, House amendments, *Congressional Record*, daily edition, February 14, 2011, pp. H776-H777. The entities listed in the amendment were the same as those on the website Planned Parenthood Federation of America, *Local & State Offices*, http://www.plannedparenthood.org/about-us/affiliate-and-state-offices.htm.

H.R. 3070, the Departments of Labor, Health and Human Services, and Education, and Related Agencies Appropriations Act, 2012, was introduced September 29, 2011. It would prohibit the act's funds from being made available "for any purpose" to PPFA or any of its affiliates and clinics, unless they certify that PPFA affiliates and clinics will not perform an abortion, and will not provide any funds to any other entity that performs an abortion. There are exceptions for rape, incest, and certain physician-certified cases where the woman is "in danger of death unless an abortion is performed." The HHS Secretary would be required to "seek repayment of any Federal assistance received by Planned Parenthood Federation of America, Inc., or any affiliate or clinic of Planned Parenthood Federation of America, Inc., if it violates the terms of the certification required by this section." H.R. 3070 was referred to the House Committee on Appropriations.

On July 18, 2012, the House Appropriations Subcommittee on Labor, Health and Human Services, Education, and Related Agencies approved a draft FY2013 Labor-HHS-Education bill.[119] The draft includes the same language as H.R. 3070 on restricting the act's funds to PPFA and its affiliates.

Maternity Care Home Demonstration

H.R. 3620/S. 1969, the Quality Care for Moms and Babies Act, would authorize a three-year Maternity Care Home Demonstration Program. Title X clinics would be eligible to participate. A maternity care home would be required to use practice innovations and coordination agreements with other providers to improve the management and coordination of maternity care for women, including family planning. H.R. 3620 was introduced December 8, 2011, and referred to the House Committee on Energy and Commerce. S. 1969 was introduced December 8, 2011, and referred to the Senate Committee on Finance.

HIV/AIDS Provider Loan Repayment Program

H.R. 6138, Ending the HIV/AIDS Epidemic Act of 2012, would authorize an educational loan repayment program for physicians, nurse practitioners, or physician assistants who serve at least two years in an area with high HIV/AIDS incidence or at a Ryan White-funded or Title X-funded facility with a critical shortage of doctors (as determined by the HHS Secretary). H.R. 6138 was introduced July 18, 2012, and referred to the House Committees on Energy and Commerce, Foreign Affairs, Education and the Workforce, Judiciary, Armed Services, Financial Services, and Ways and Means.

---

[119] U.S. Congress, House Committee on Appropriations, Subcommittee on Labor, Health and Human Services, Education, and Related Agencies, *Making appropriations for the Departments of Labor, Health and Human Services, and Education, and related agencies for the fiscal year ending September 30, 2012, and for other purposes*, Draft bill, 112th Cong., 2nd sess., July 15, 2012, Sec. 536, pp. 146-147, http://appropriations.house.gov/uploadedfiles/bills-112hr-sc-ap-fy13-laborhhsed.pdf.

Appendix. Summary of Title X of the Public Health Service Act

Below is a summary of Title X of the Public Health Service Act, codified at 42 U.S.C. Section 300 to Section 300a-6, Population Research and Voluntary Family Planning Programs:

Section 1001. Project Grants and Contracts for Family Planning Services

The Secretary may make grants to and enter into contracts with public or nonprofit private entities to assist in the establishment and operation of voluntary family planning projects to offer a broad range of acceptable and effective family planning methods and services (including natural family planning methods, infertility services, and services for adolescents). Entities which receive grants or contracts must encourage family participation in their projects.

Section 1002. Formula Grants to States for Family Planning Services[120]

The Secretary may make grants to state health authorities to assist in planning, establishing, maintaining, coordinating, and evaluating family planning services. The state health authority must have an approved state plan for a coordinated and comprehensive program of family planning services.

Section 1003. Training Grants and Contracts

The Secretary may make grants to public or nonprofit private entities and enter into contracts with public or private entities and individuals to provide the training for personnel to carry out family planning service programs.

Section 1004. Research

The Secretary may conduct and make grants to public or nonprofit private entities and enter into contracts with public or private entities and individuals for projects for research in the biomedical, contraceptive development, behavioral, and program implementation fields related to family planning and population.

Section 1005. Informational and Educational Materials

The Secretary may make grants to public or nonprofit private entities and enter into contracts with public or private entities and individuals to assist in developing and making available family

---

[120] These formula grants, which were authorized for FY1971-FY1973, were never funded. S.Rept. 101-95, pp. 5, 10.

planning and population growth information (including educational materials) to all persons desiring such information.

Section 1006. Regulations and Payments

The Secretary may promulgate regulations and must determine the conditions for making payments to grantees to assure that such grants will be effectively utilized for the purposes they were made.

Grantees must assure that (1) priority will be given to the furnishing of services to persons from low-income families; and (2) no charge will be made in such project or program for services provided to any person from a low-income family except to the extent that payment will be made by a third party (including a government agency) which is authorized or is under legal obligation to pay the charge.

The Secretary must be satisfied that informational or educational materials developed or made available under the grant or contract will be suitable for the purposes of this title and for the population or community to which they are to be made available.

In the case of any grant or contract under Section 1001, such assurances shall provide for the review and approval of the suitability of such materials, prior to their distribution, by an advisory committee established by the grantee or contractor in accordance with regulations.

Section 1007. Voluntary Participation

The acceptance by any individual of family planning services or family planning or population growth information (including educational materials) shall be voluntary and shall not be a prerequisite to eligibility for or receipt of any other service or assistance from, or to participation in, any other program of the entity or individual that provided such service or information.

Section 1008. Prohibition of Abortion

None of the funds appropriated under this title shall be used in programs where abortion is a method of family planning.

Author Contact Information

Angela Napili
Information Research Specialist
anapili@crs.loc.gov, 7-0135

www.ingramcontent.com/pod-product-compliance
Lightning Source LLC
Chambersburg PA
CBHW081246180526

45171CB00005B/556